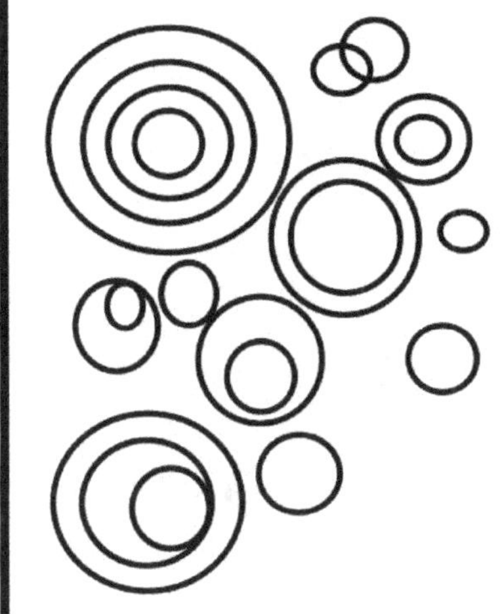

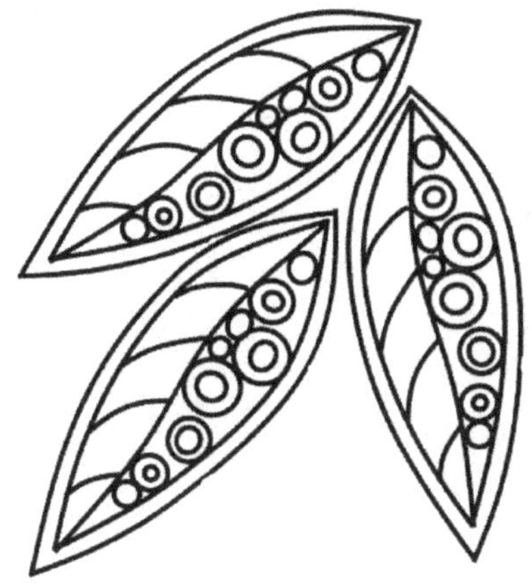

This book belongs to :

____

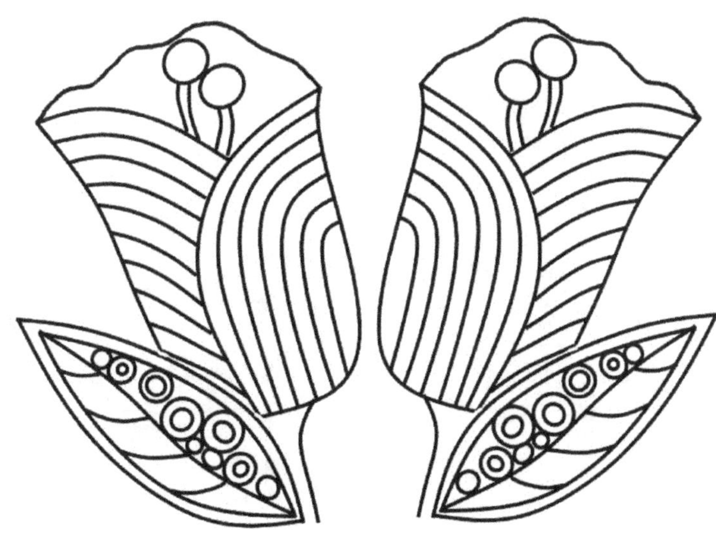

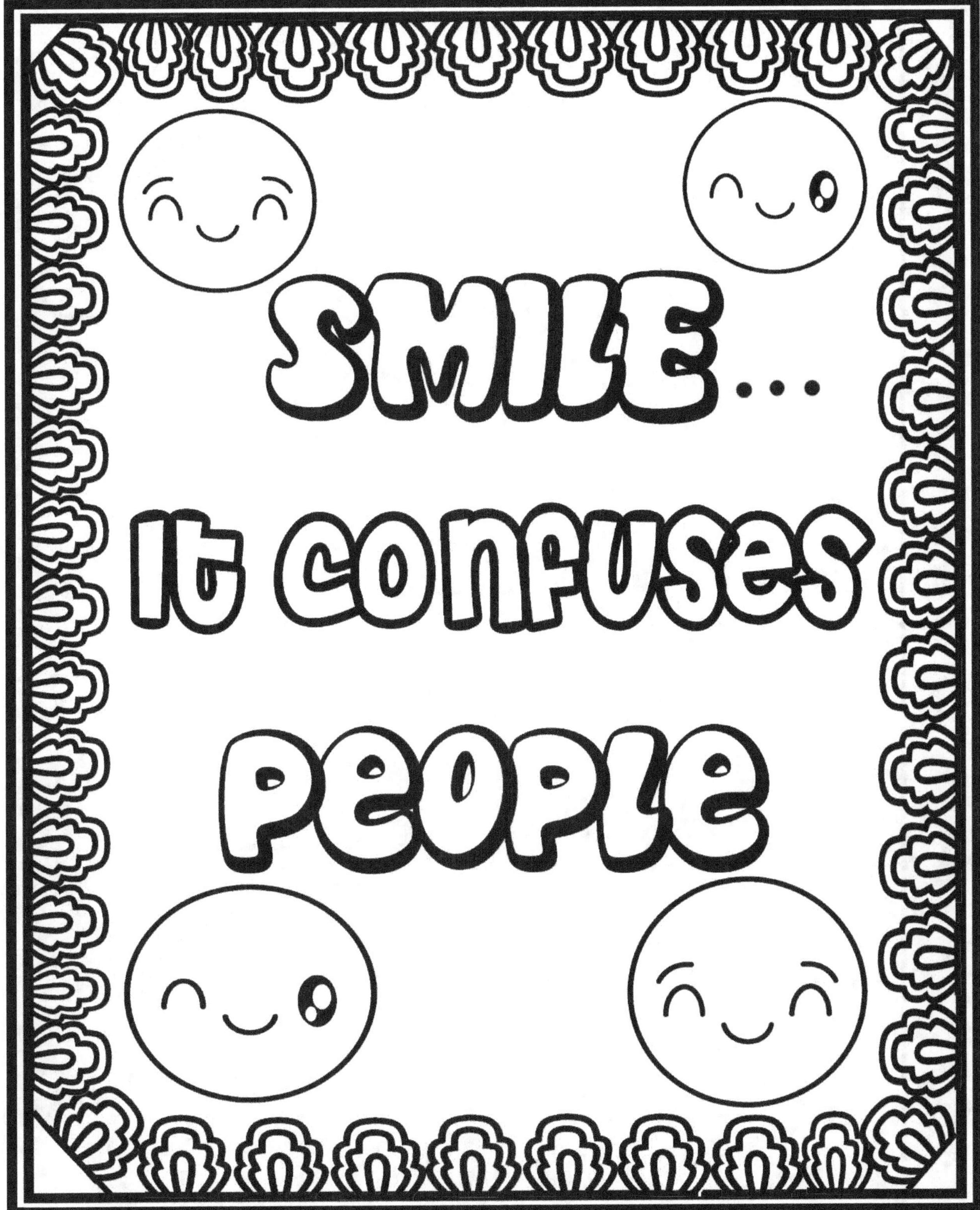

SMILE...
It confuses
PEOPLE

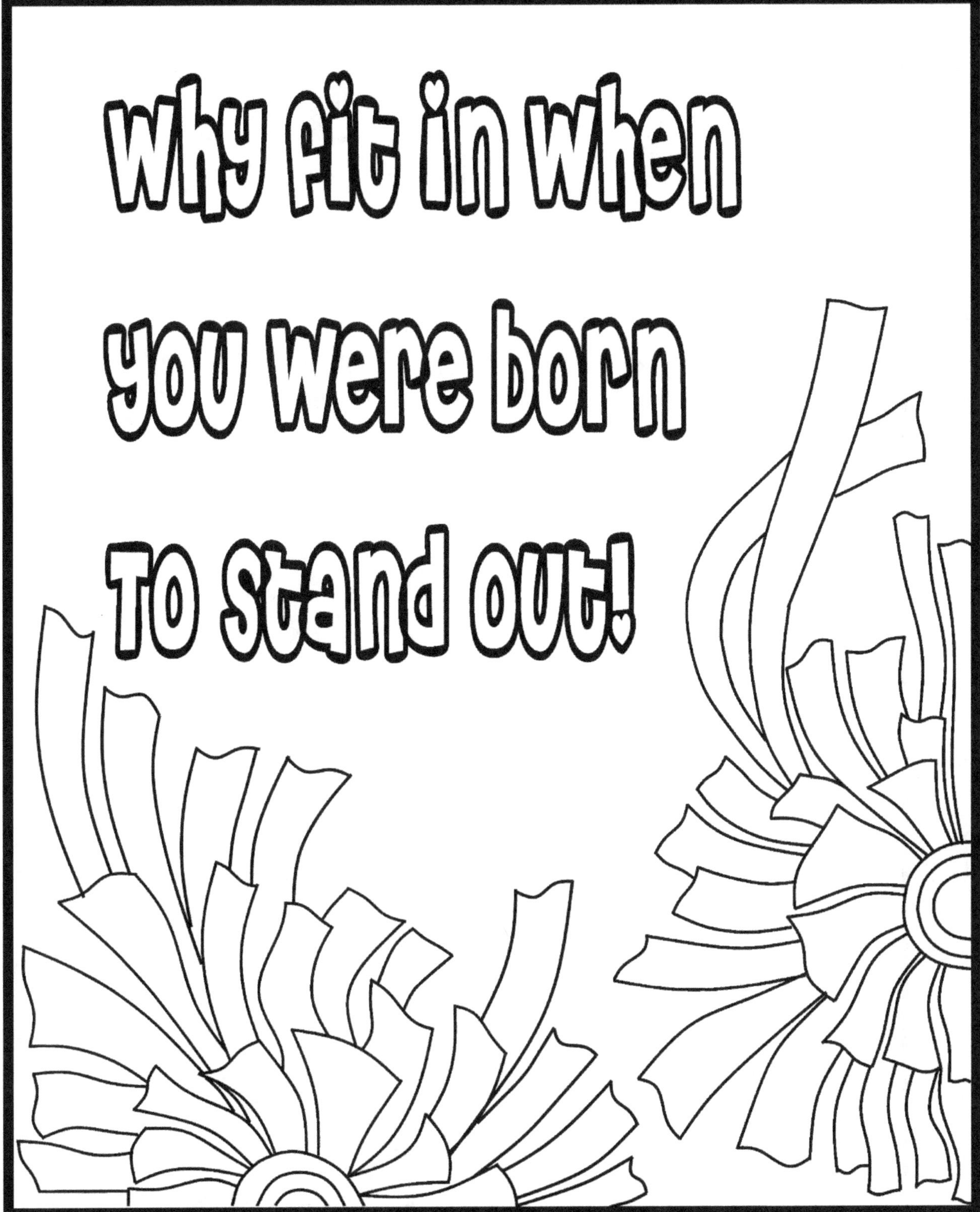

why fit in when
you were born
to stand out!

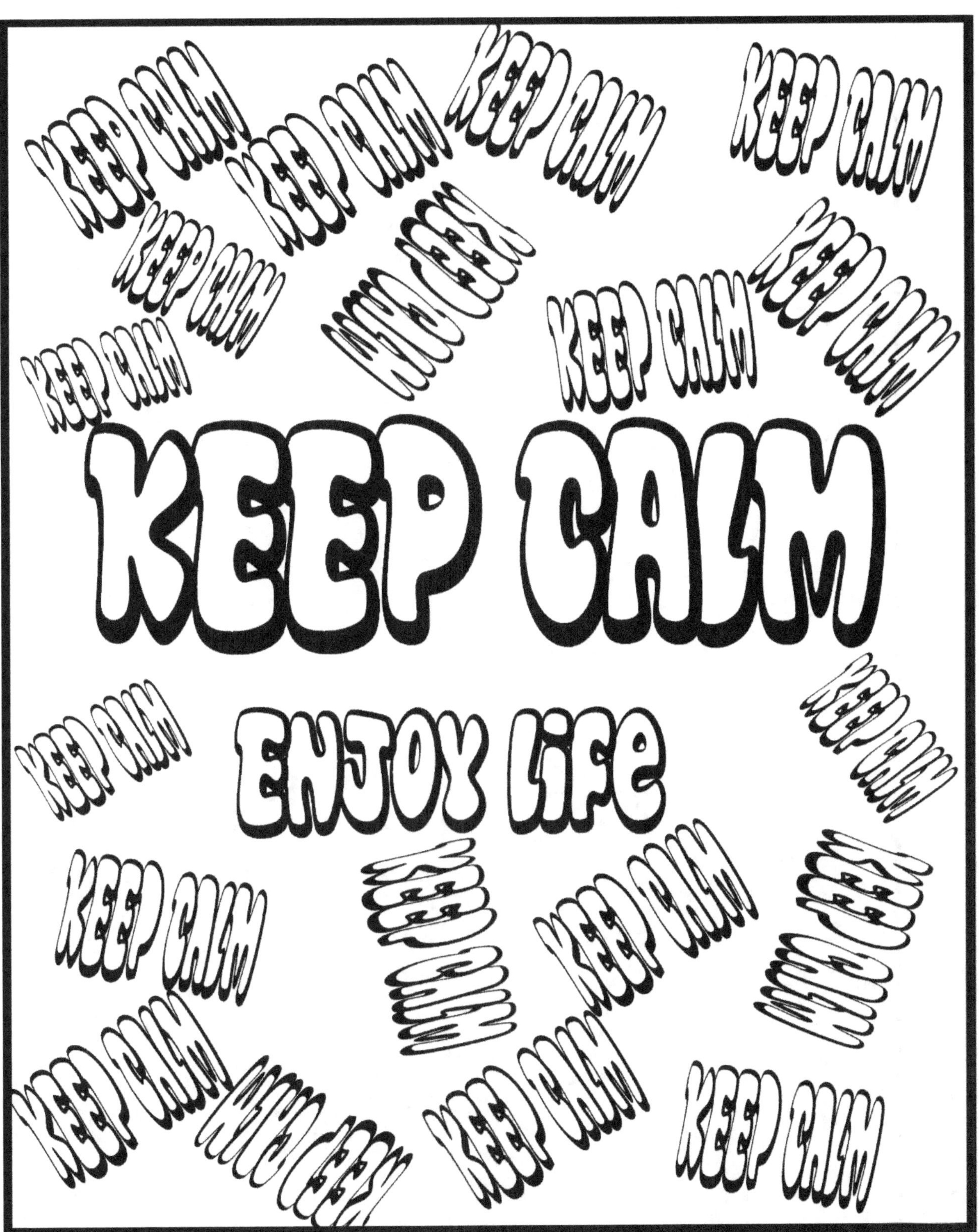

KEEP CALM
KEEP CALM
KEEP CALM
KEEP CALM
KEEP CALM
KEEP CALM
KEEP CALM
KEEP CALM
KEEP CALM
KEEP CALM
KEEP CALM
ENJOY LIFE
KEEP CALM
KEEP CALM
KEEP CALM
KEEP CALM
KEEP CALM
KEEP CALM
KEEP CALM
KEEP CALM
KEEP CALM
KEEP CALM
KEEP CALM

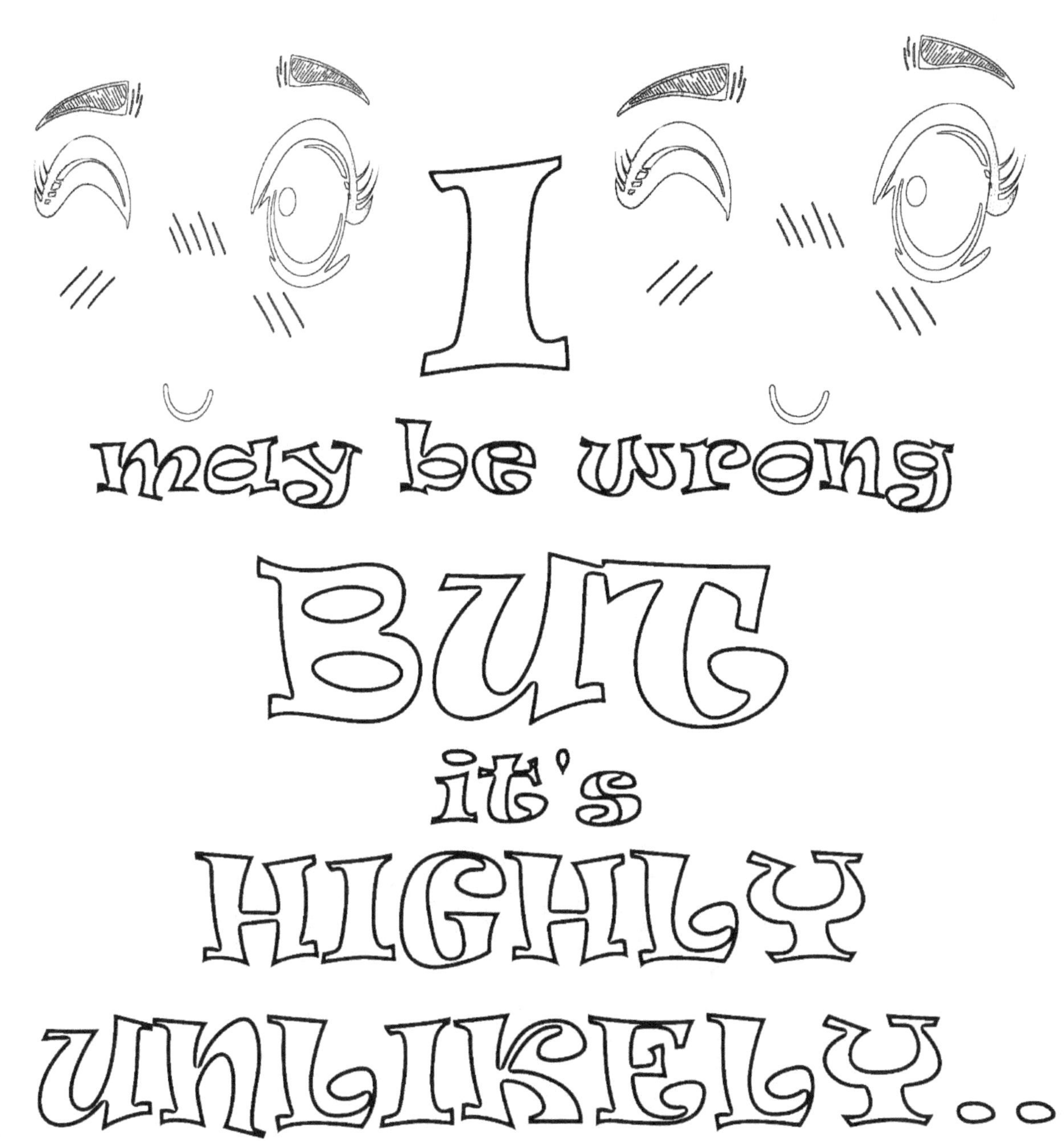
I
may be wrong
BUT
it's
HIGHLY
UNLIKELY..

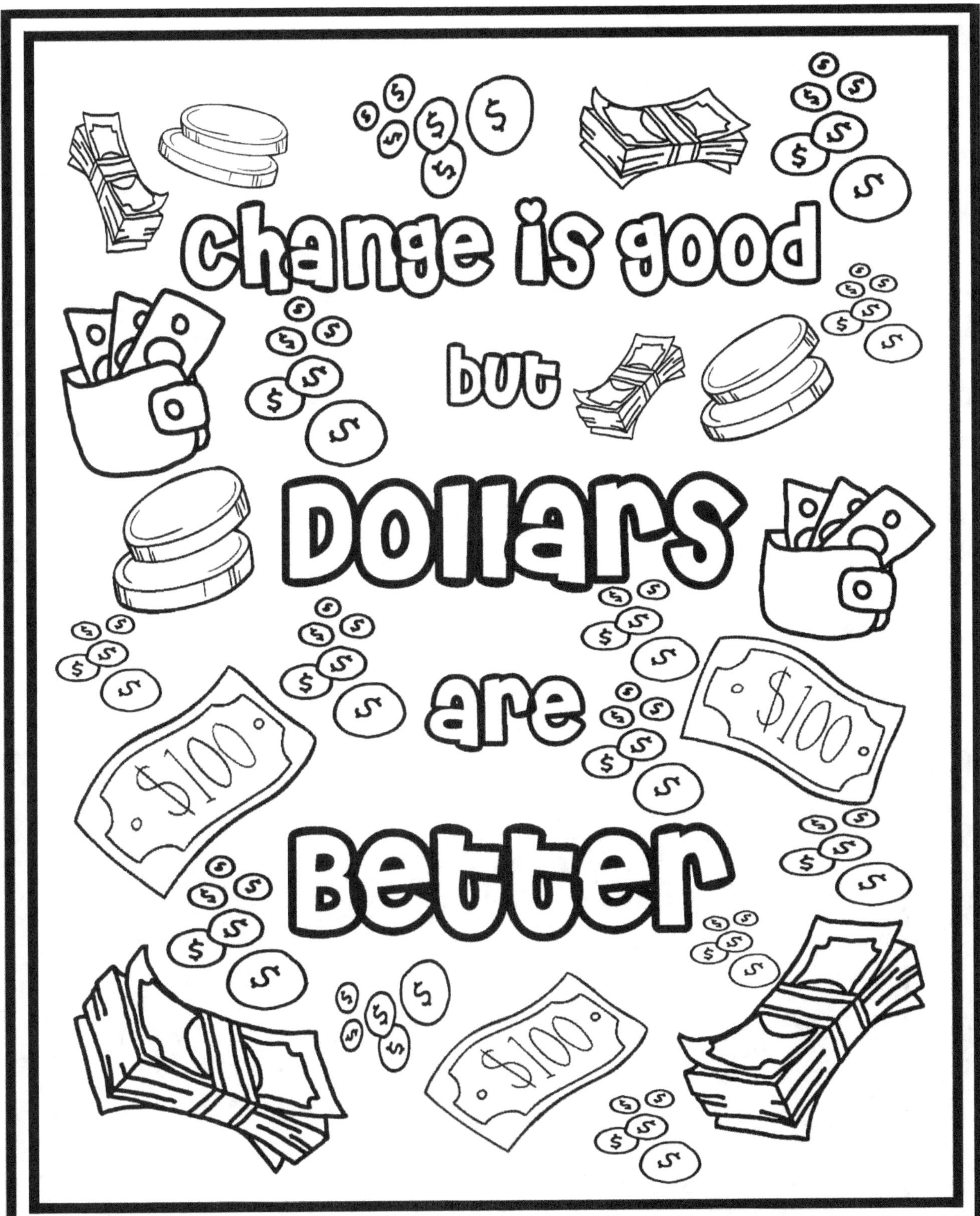

change is good
but
Dollars
are
Better
$100
$100
$100

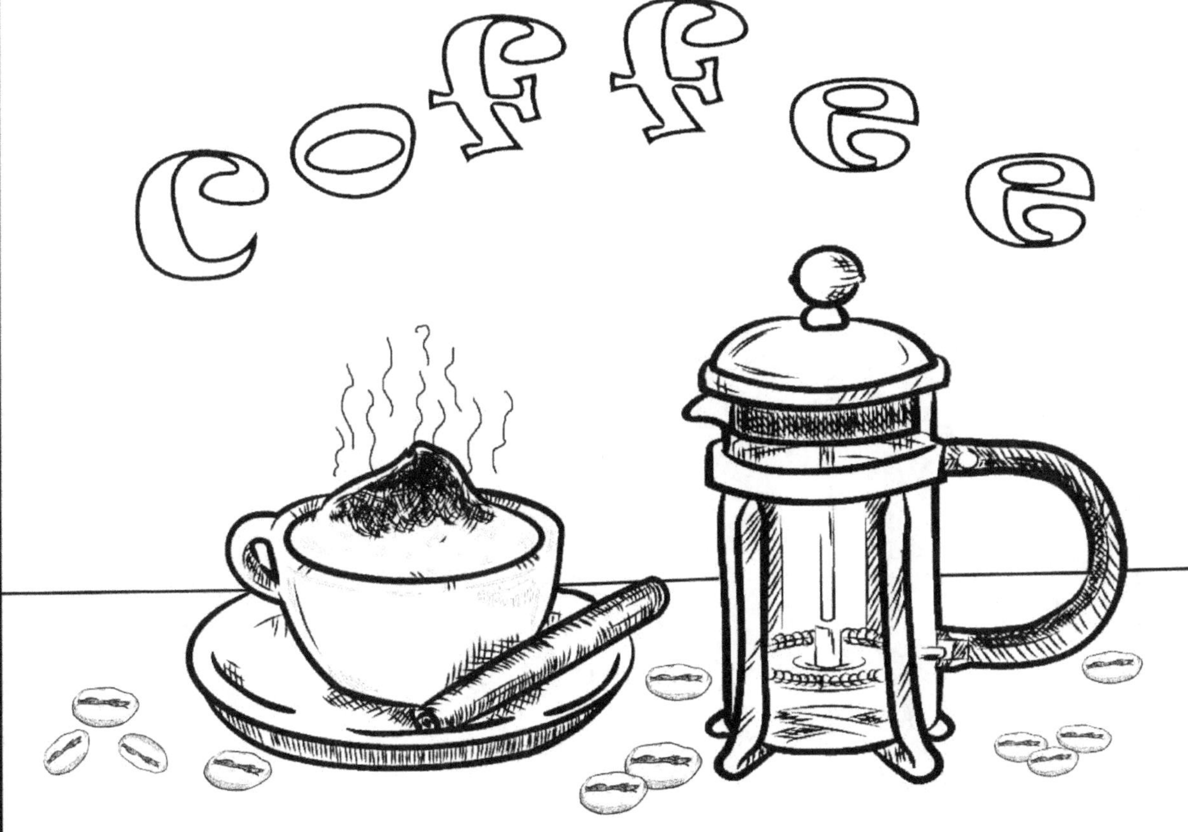

my
blood type
is
coffee

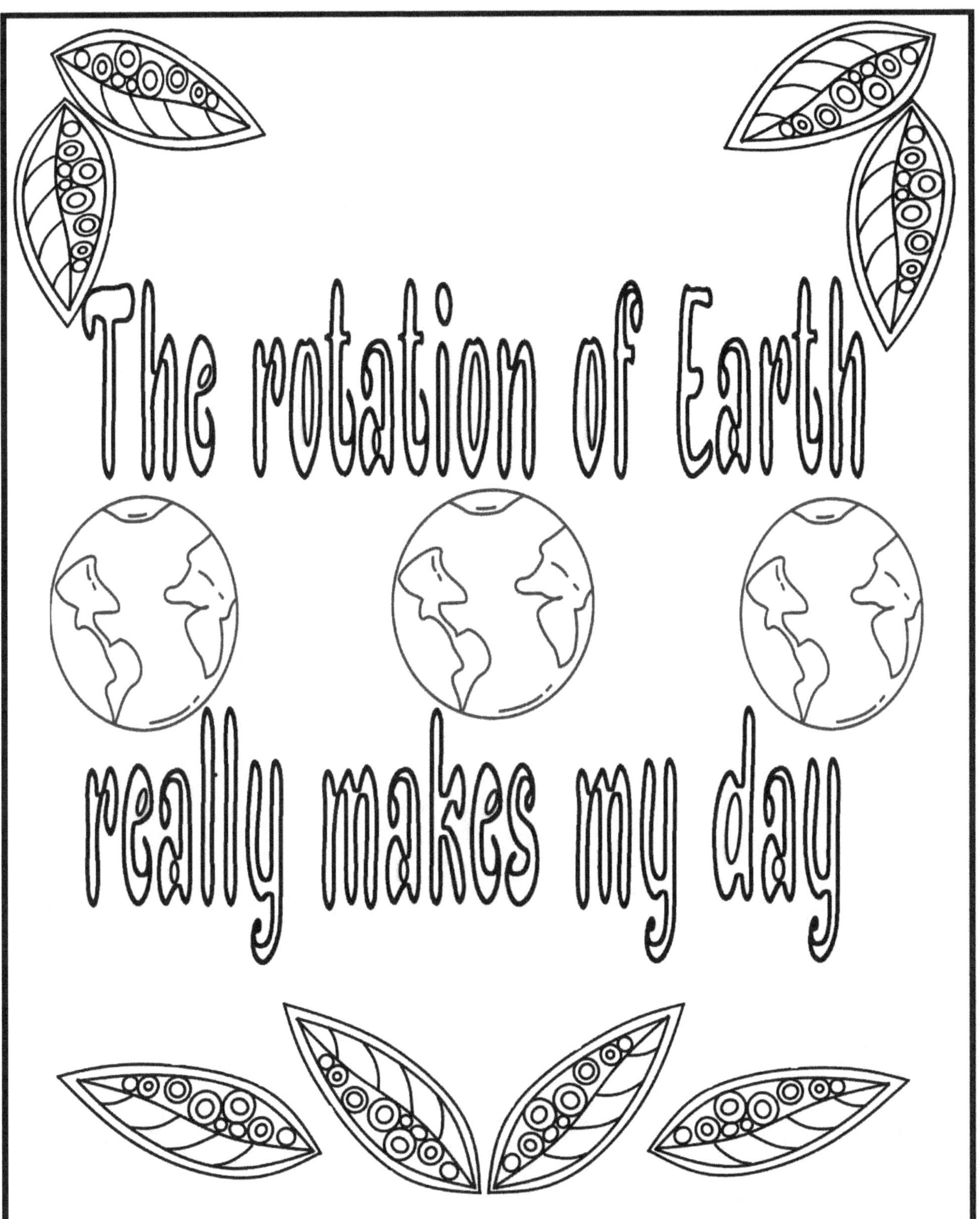

The rotation of Earth
really makes my day

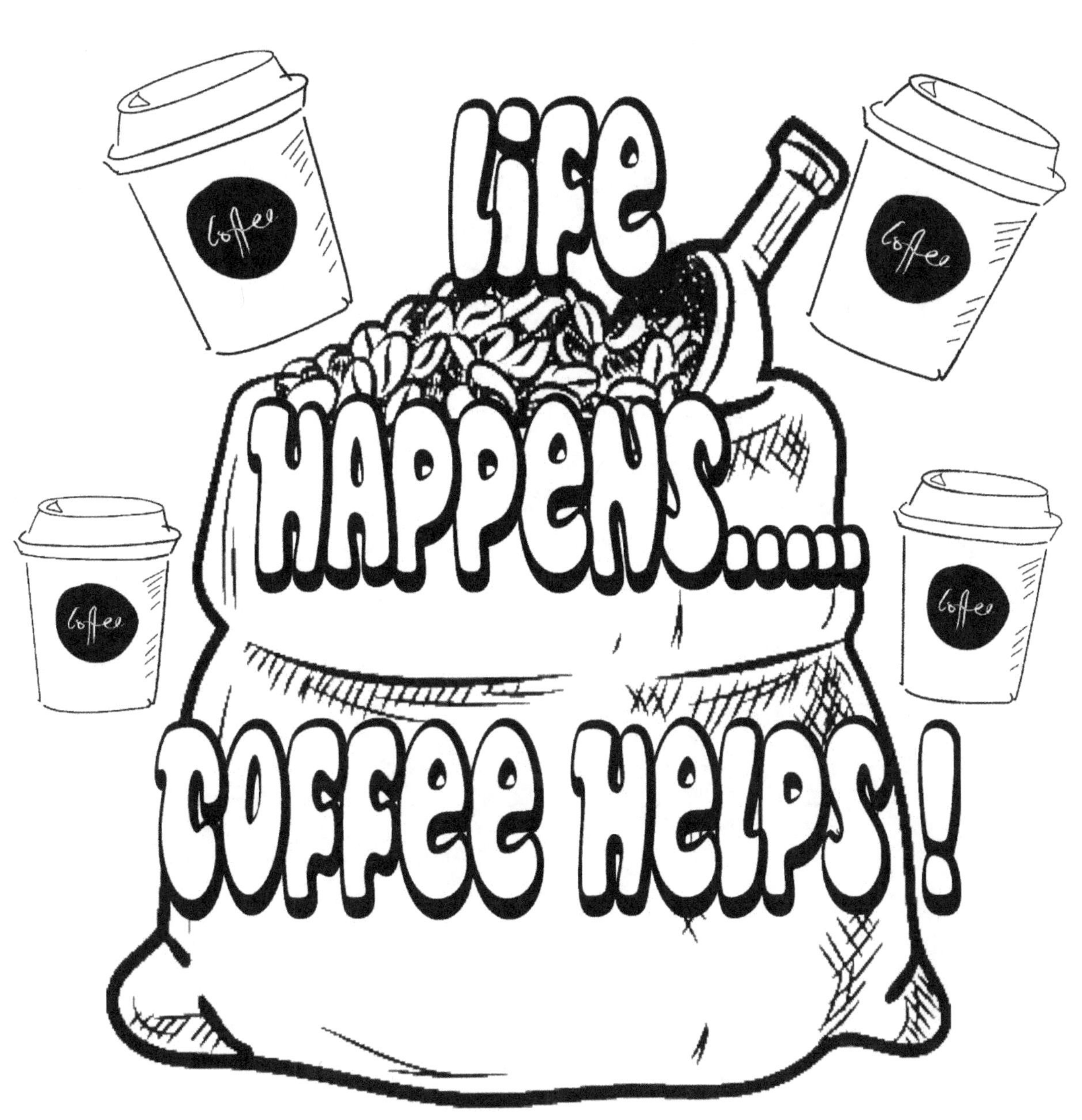

Life
HAPPENS......
COFFEE HELPS !
Coffee
Coffee
Coffee
Coffee

Do Good
and Good
will
come to
you

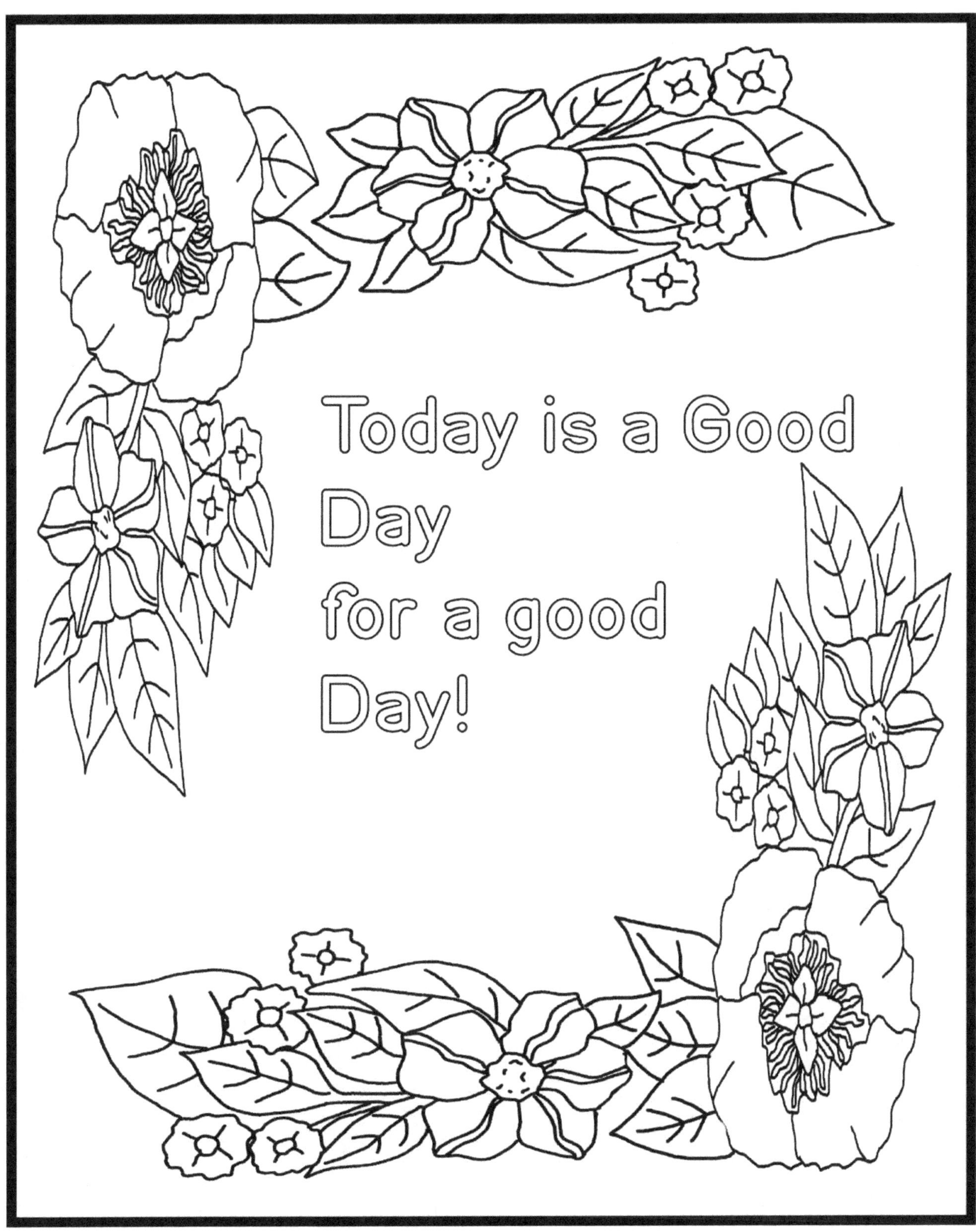

Today is a Good
Day
for a good
Day!

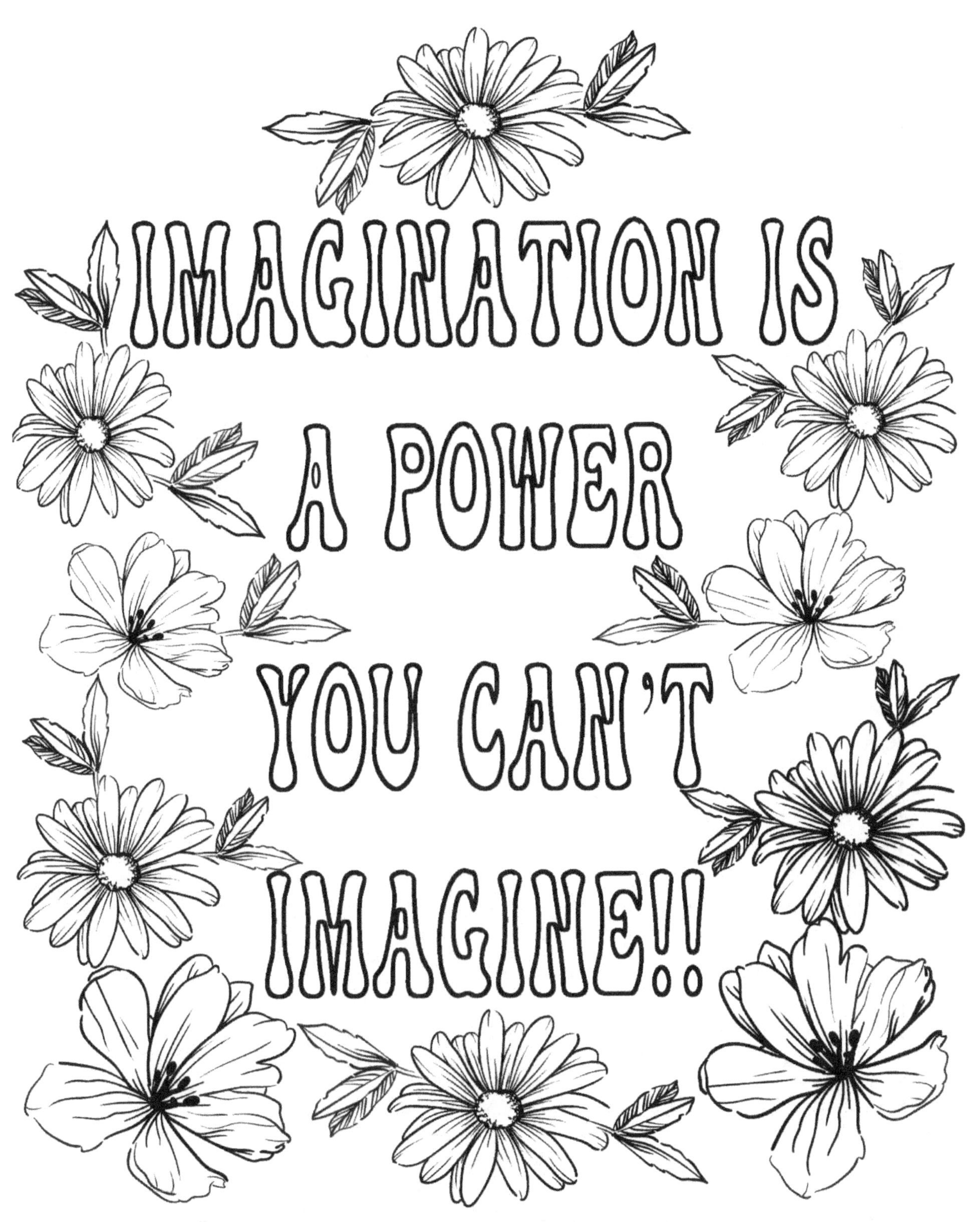

IMAGINATION IS
A POWER
YOU CAN'T
IMAGINE!!

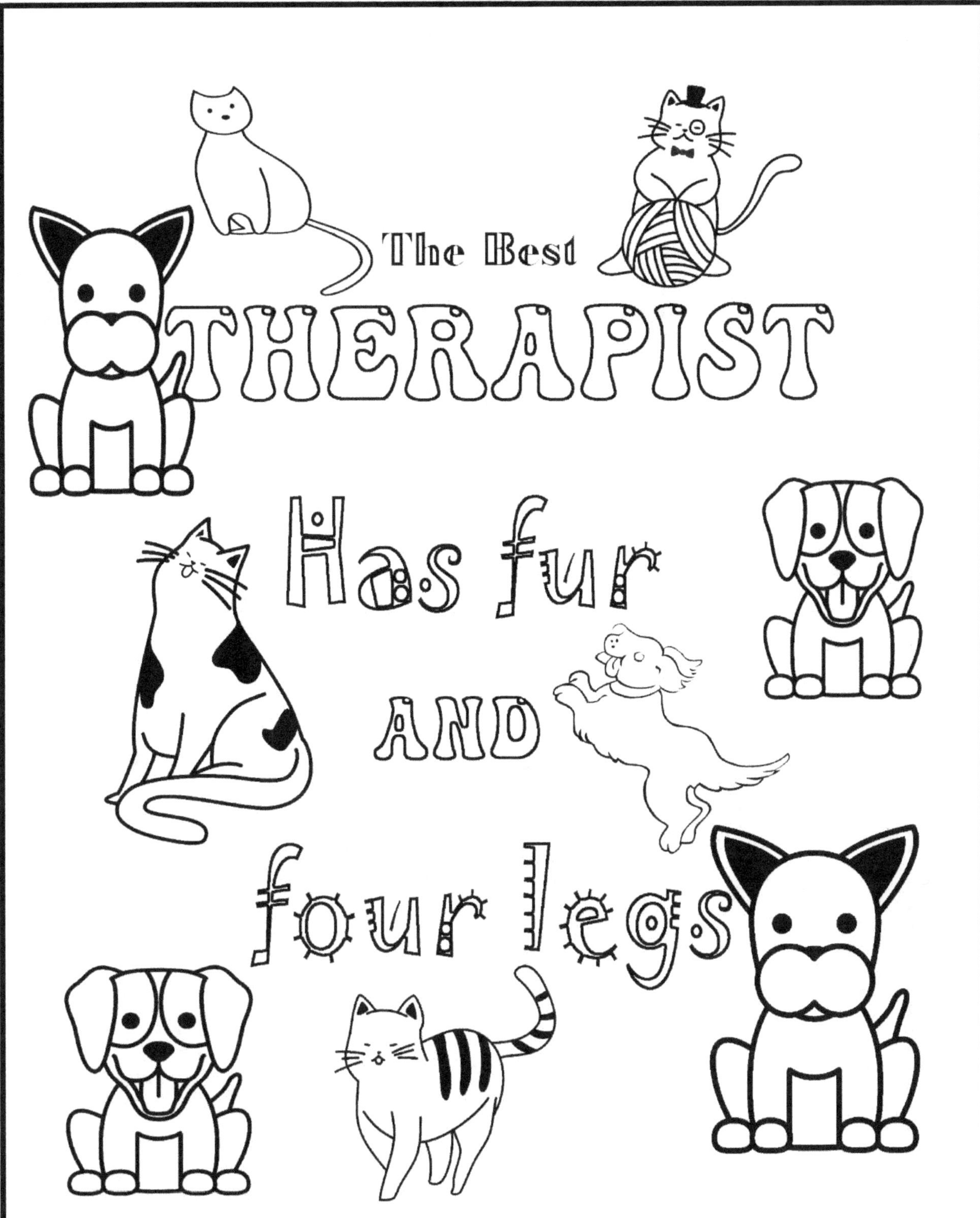

The Best
THERAPIST
Has fur
AND
four legs

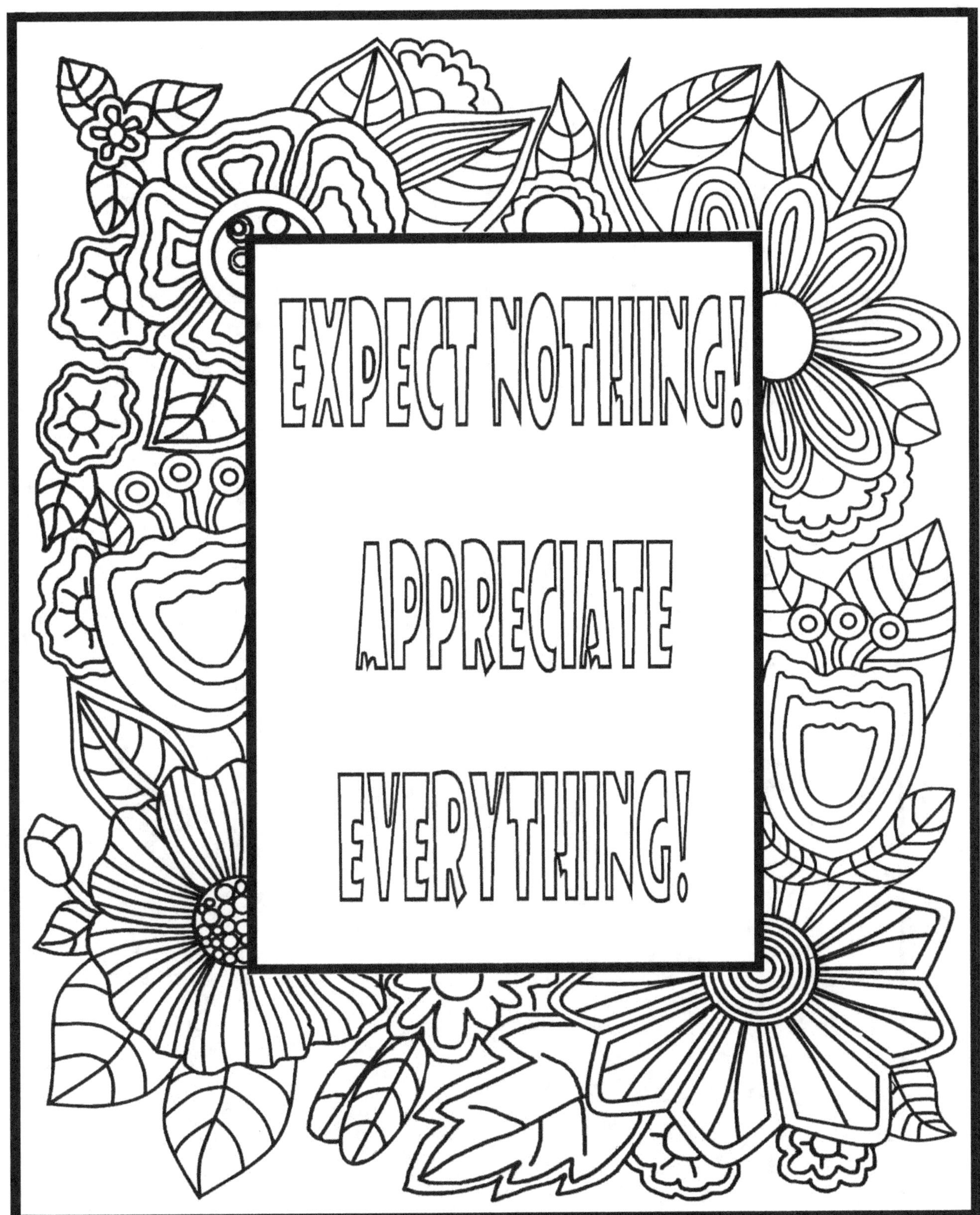

EXPECT NOTHING!
APPRECIATE
EVERYTHING!

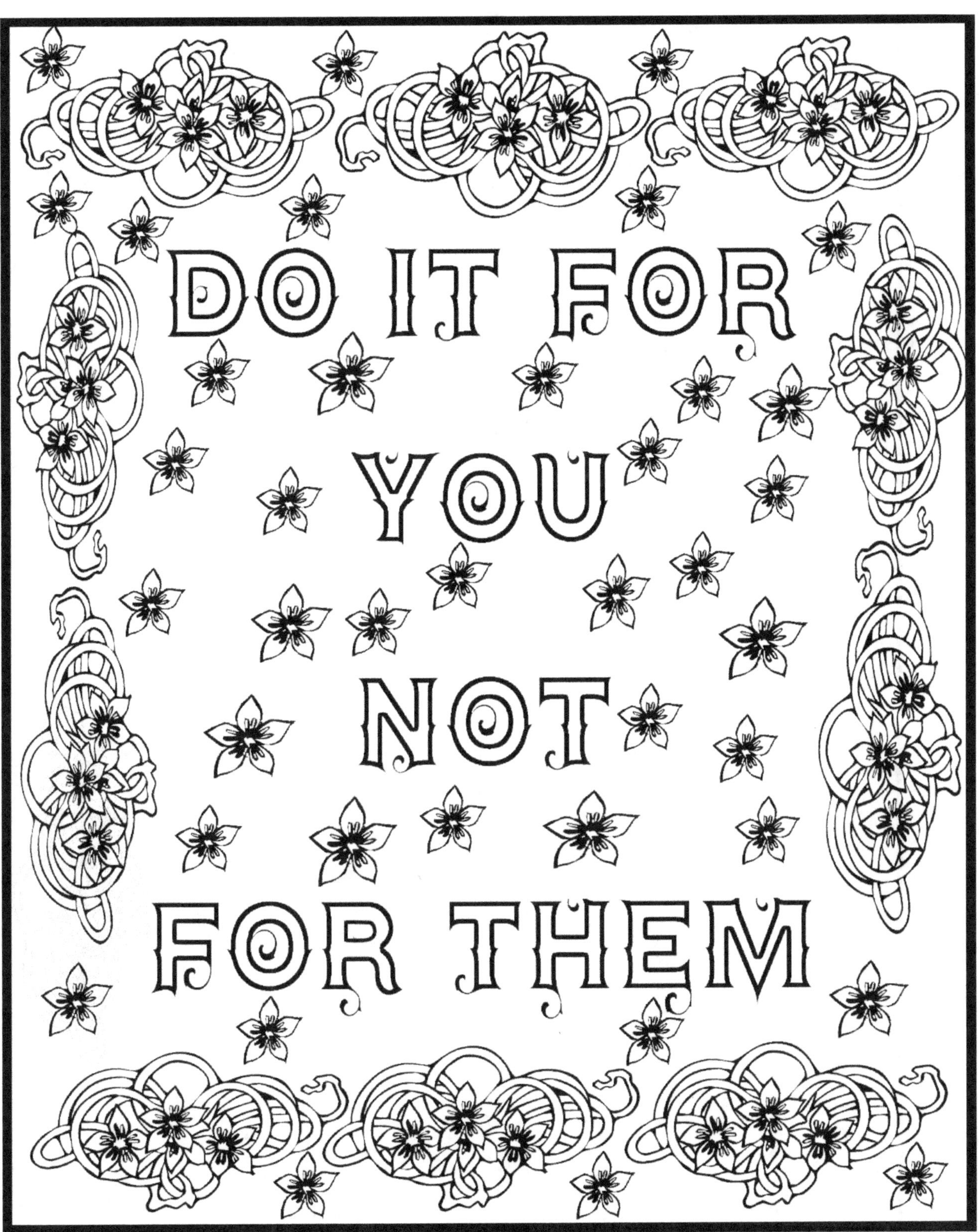

DO IT FOR
YOU
NOT
FOR THEM

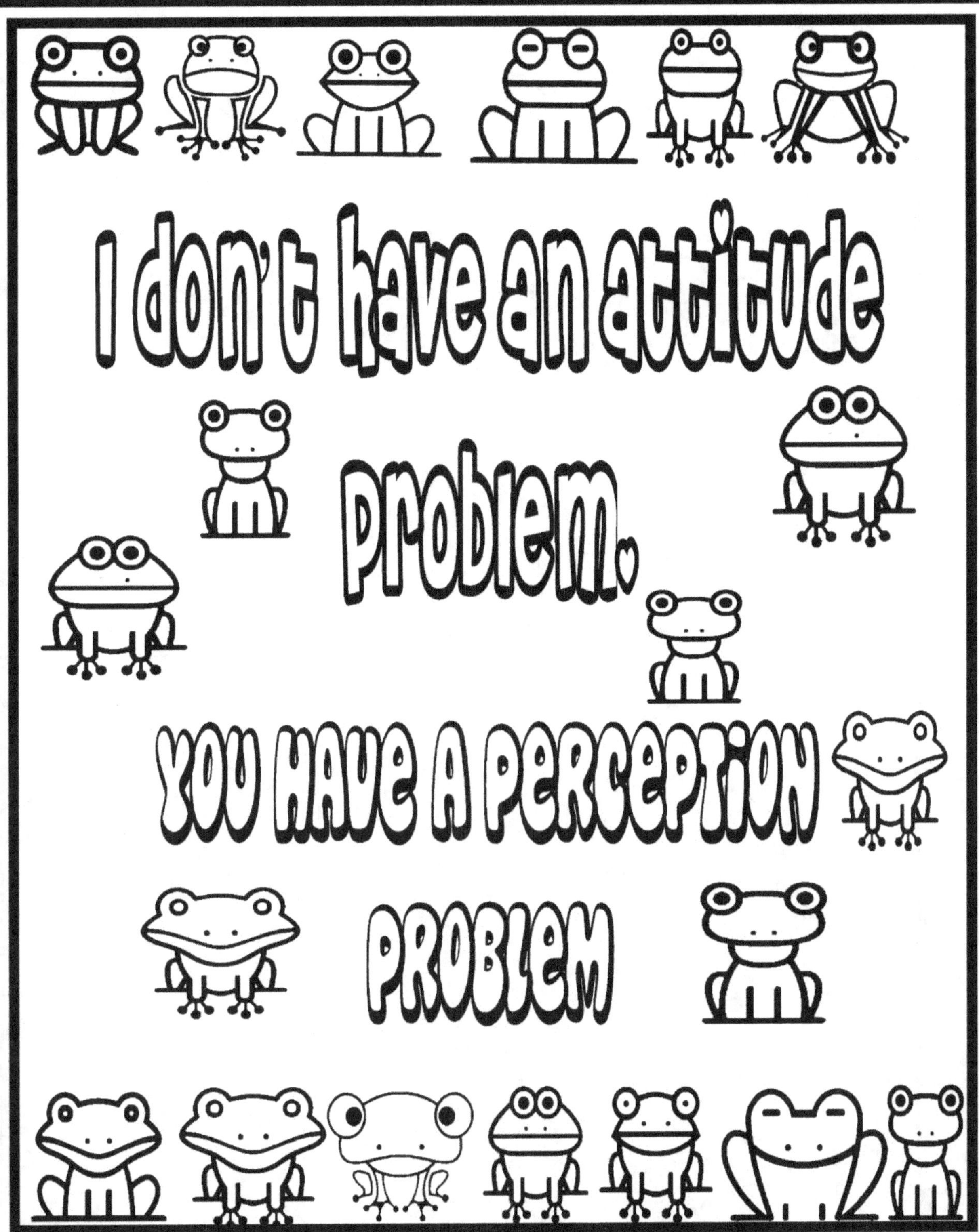

I don't have an attitude problem.
you have a perception problem

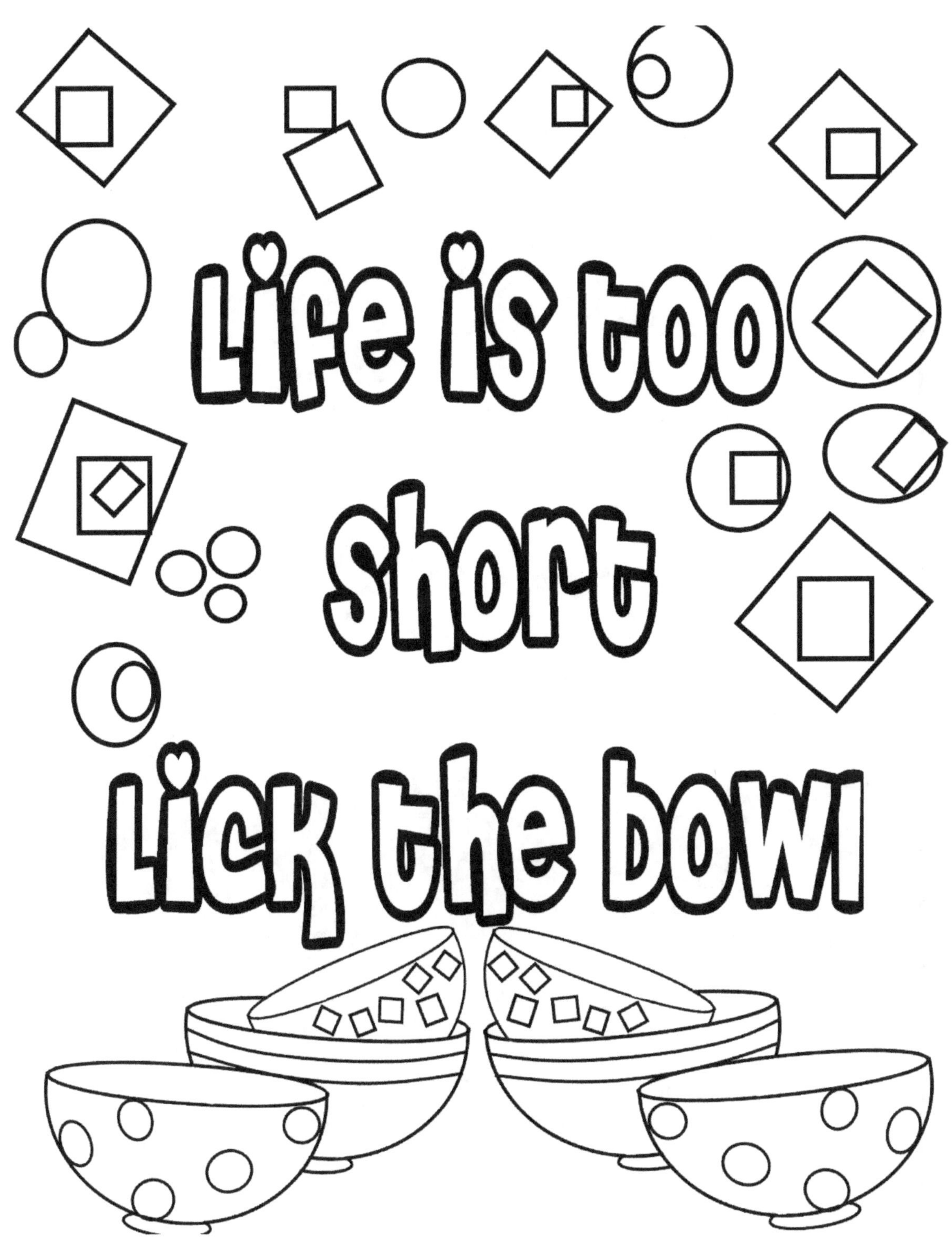

Life is too
short
Lick the bowl

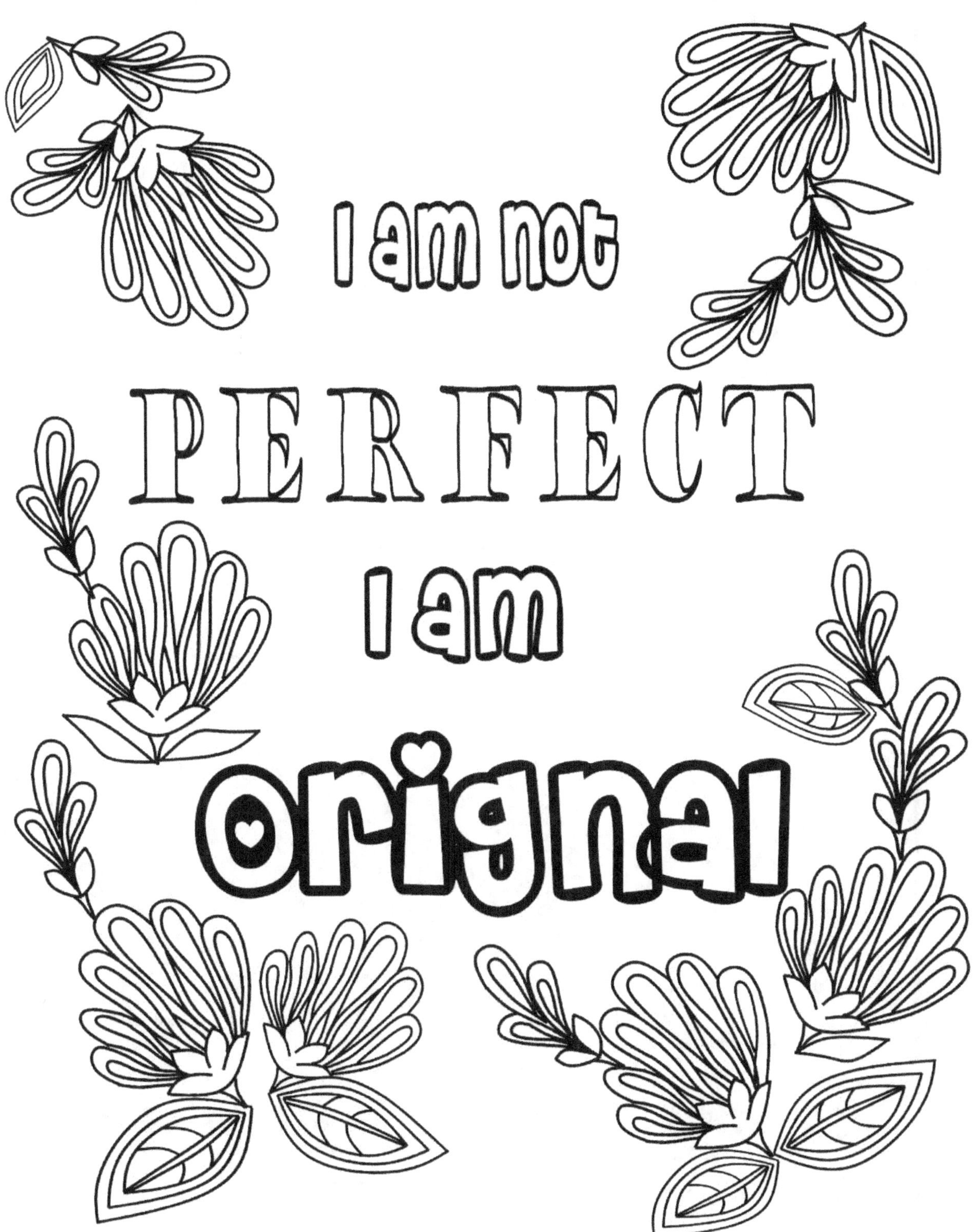

I am not
PERFECT
I am
Orignal

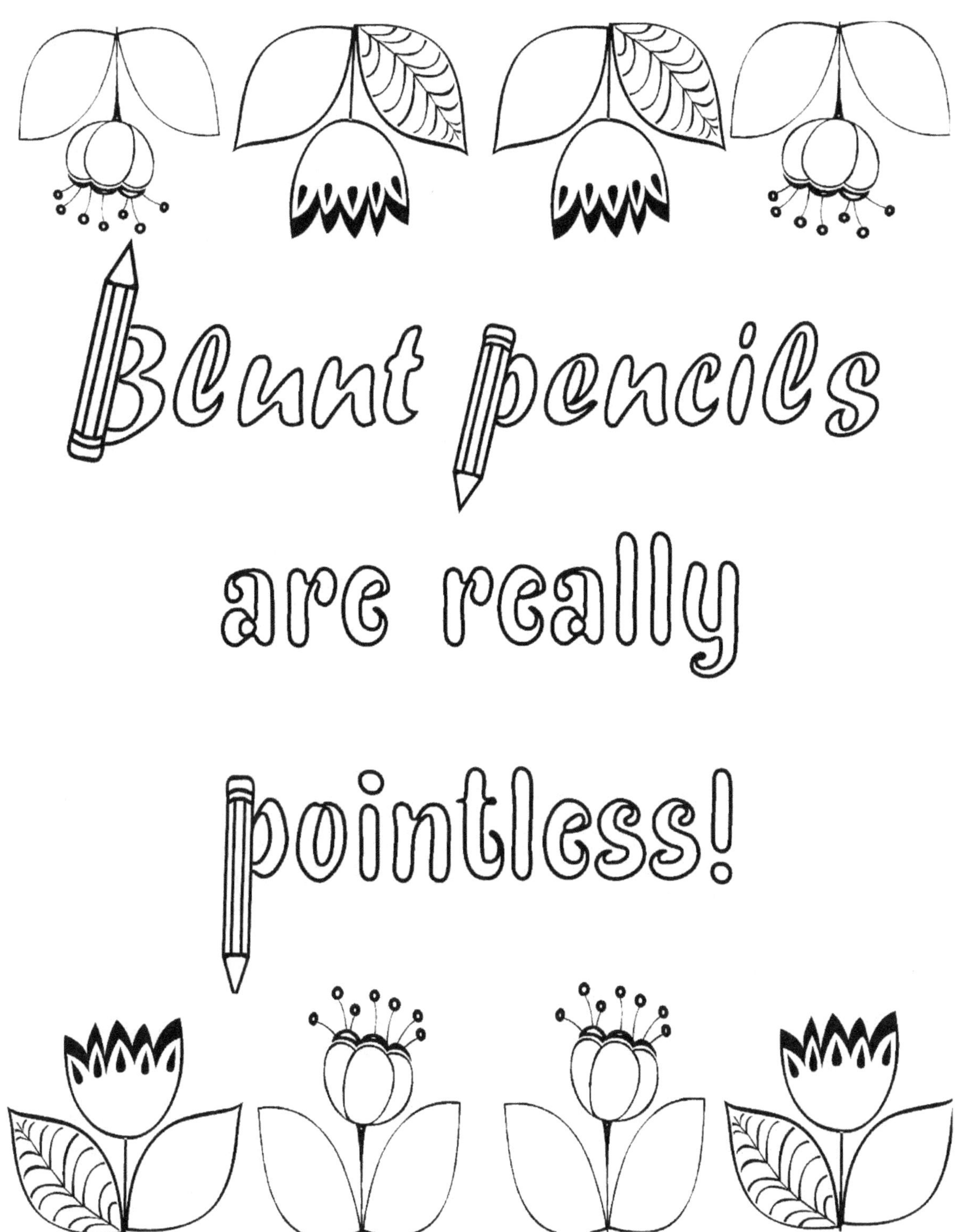

Blunt pencils
are really
pointless!

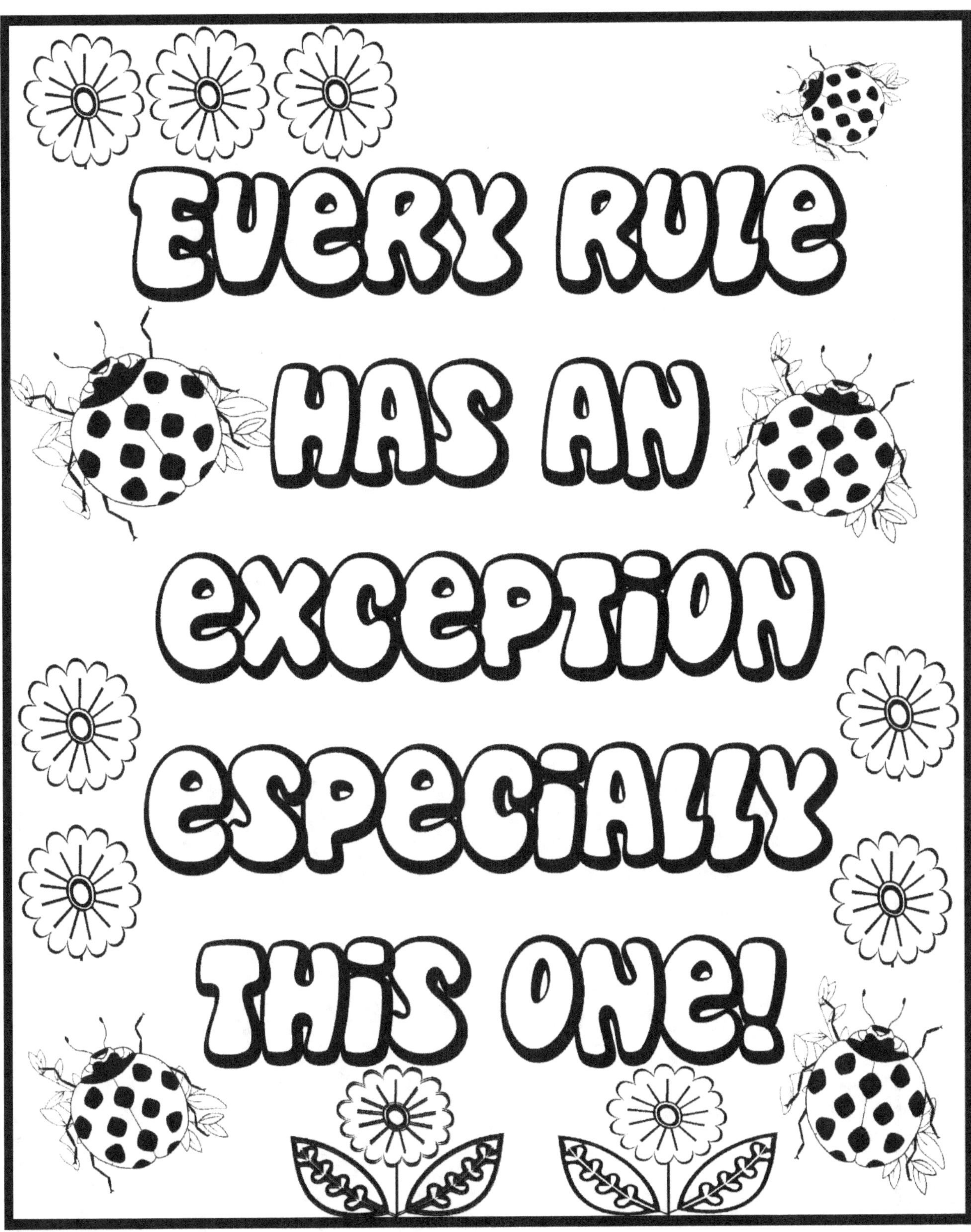

EVERY RULE
HAS AN
EXCEPTION
ESPECIALLY
THIS ONE!

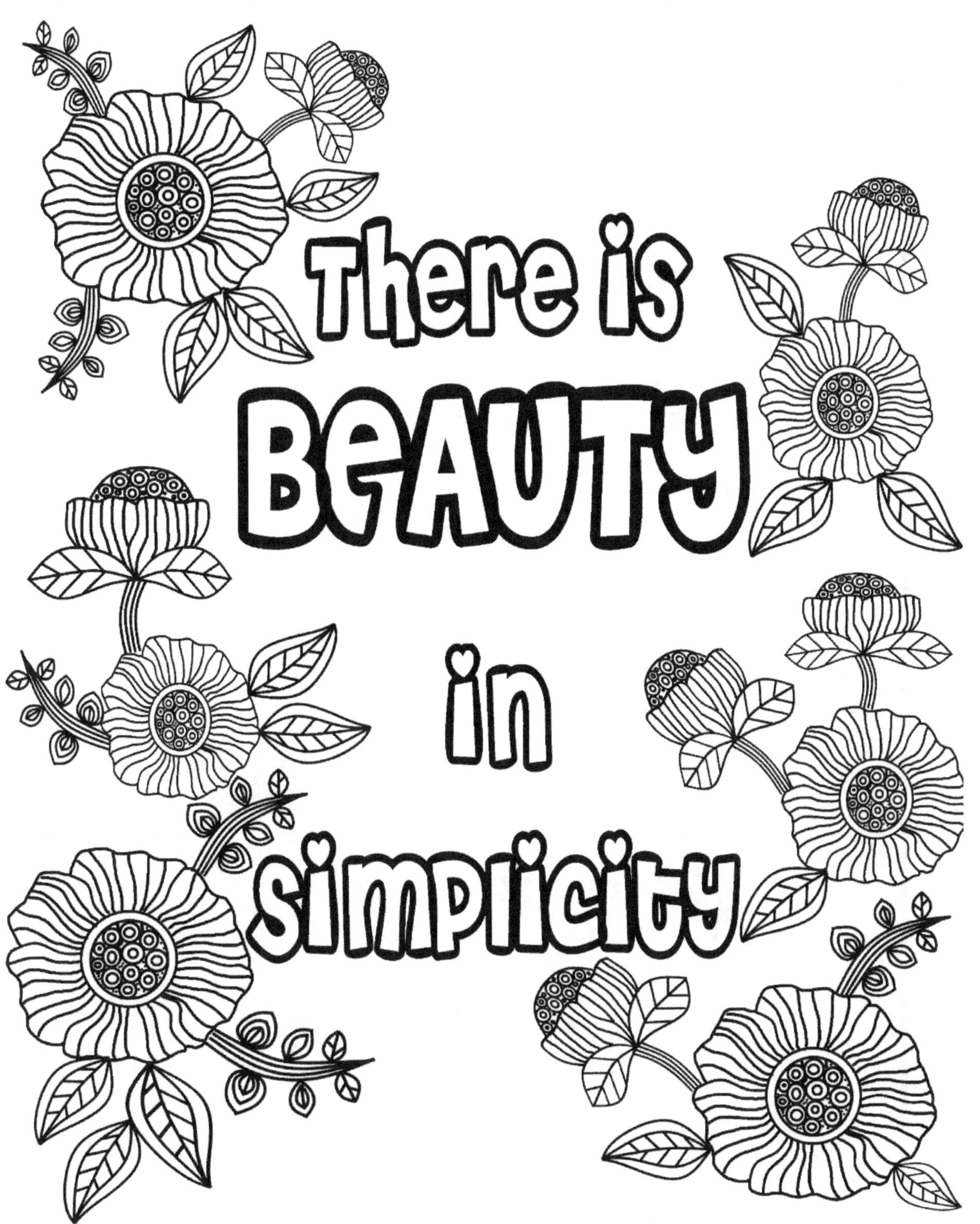

There is
BEAUTY
in
simplicity

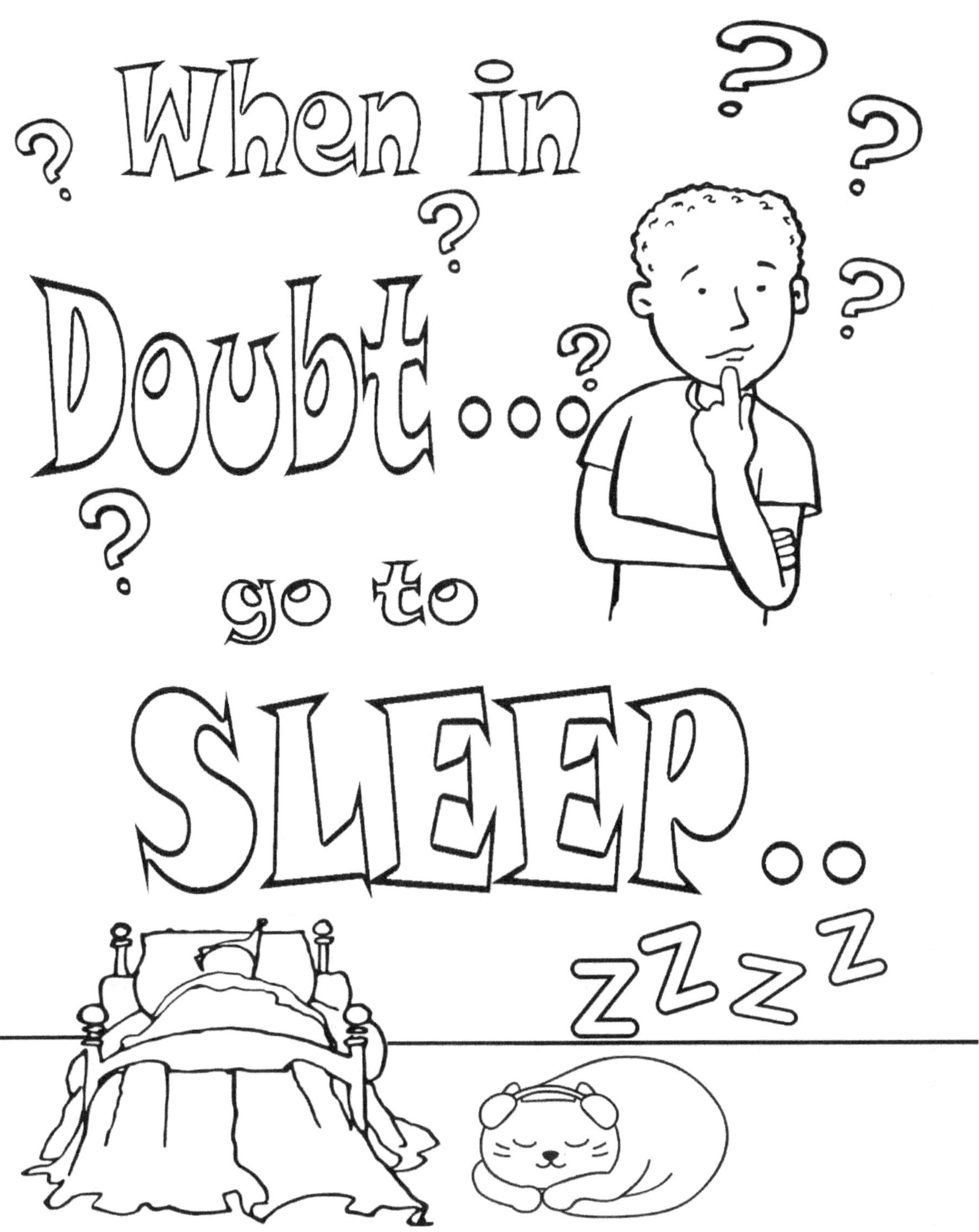

When in Doubt... go to SLEEP...
?
zzzz

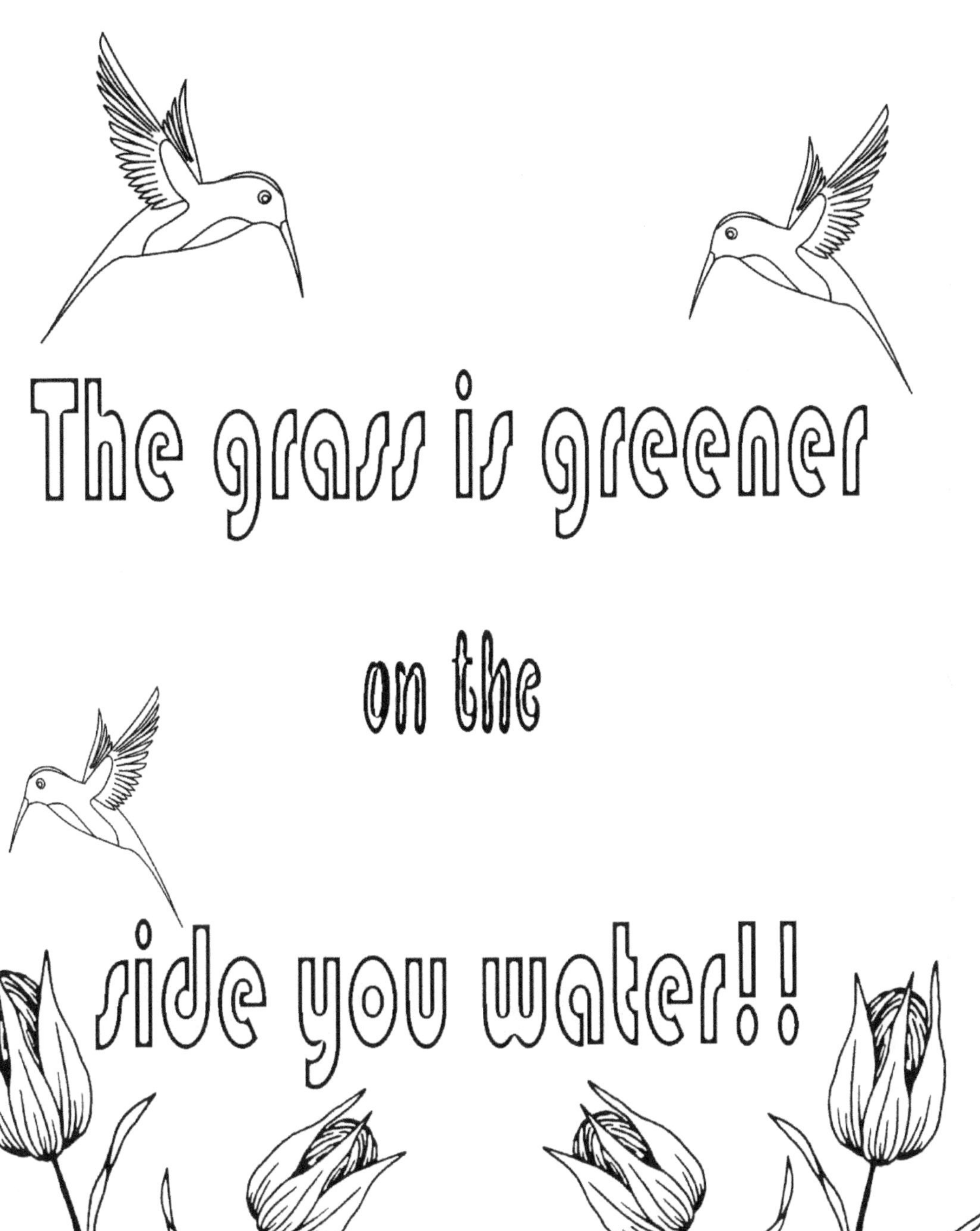

The grass is greener
on the
side you water!!

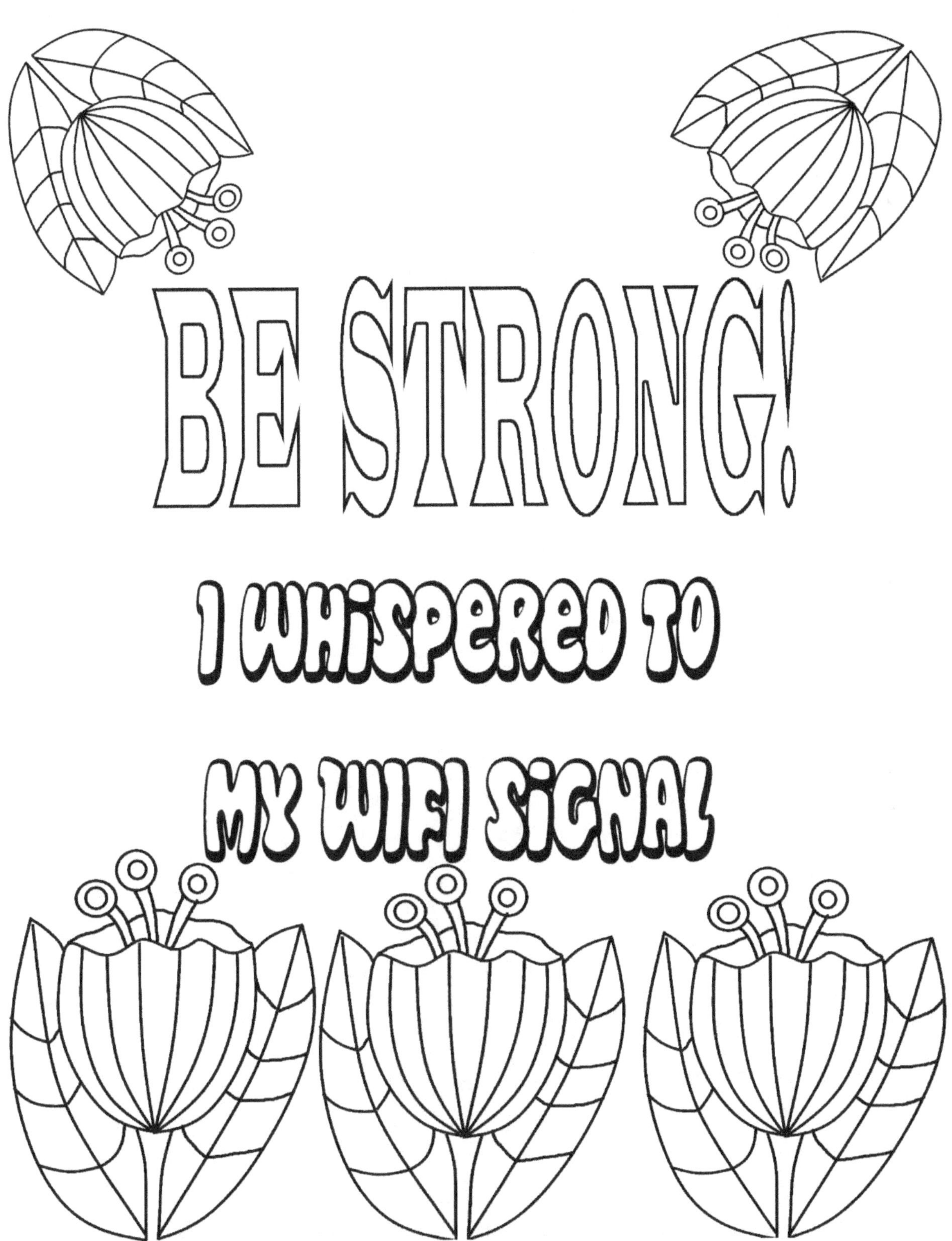
BE STRONG!
I WHISPERED TO
MY WIFI SIGNAL

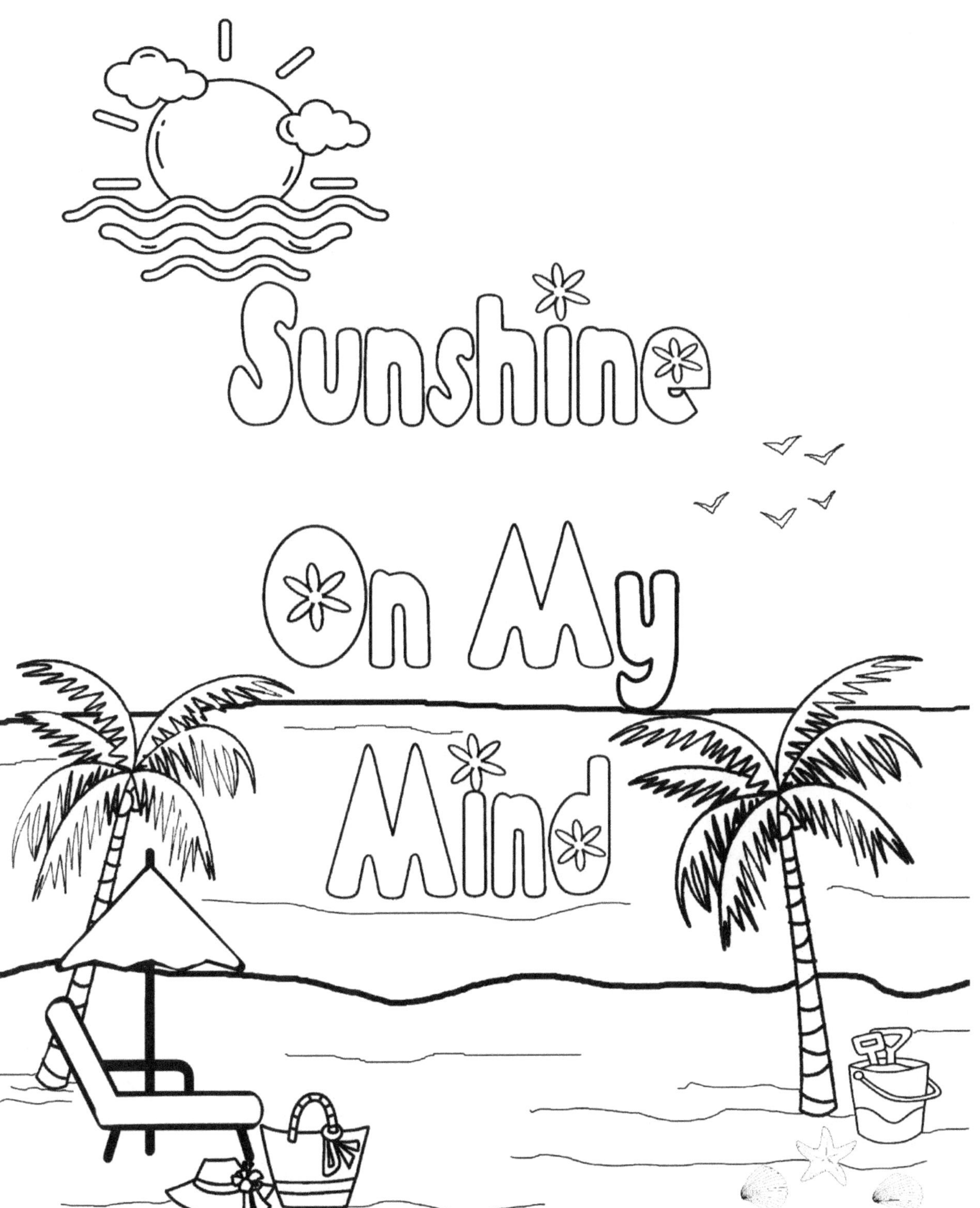

Sunshine
On My
Mind

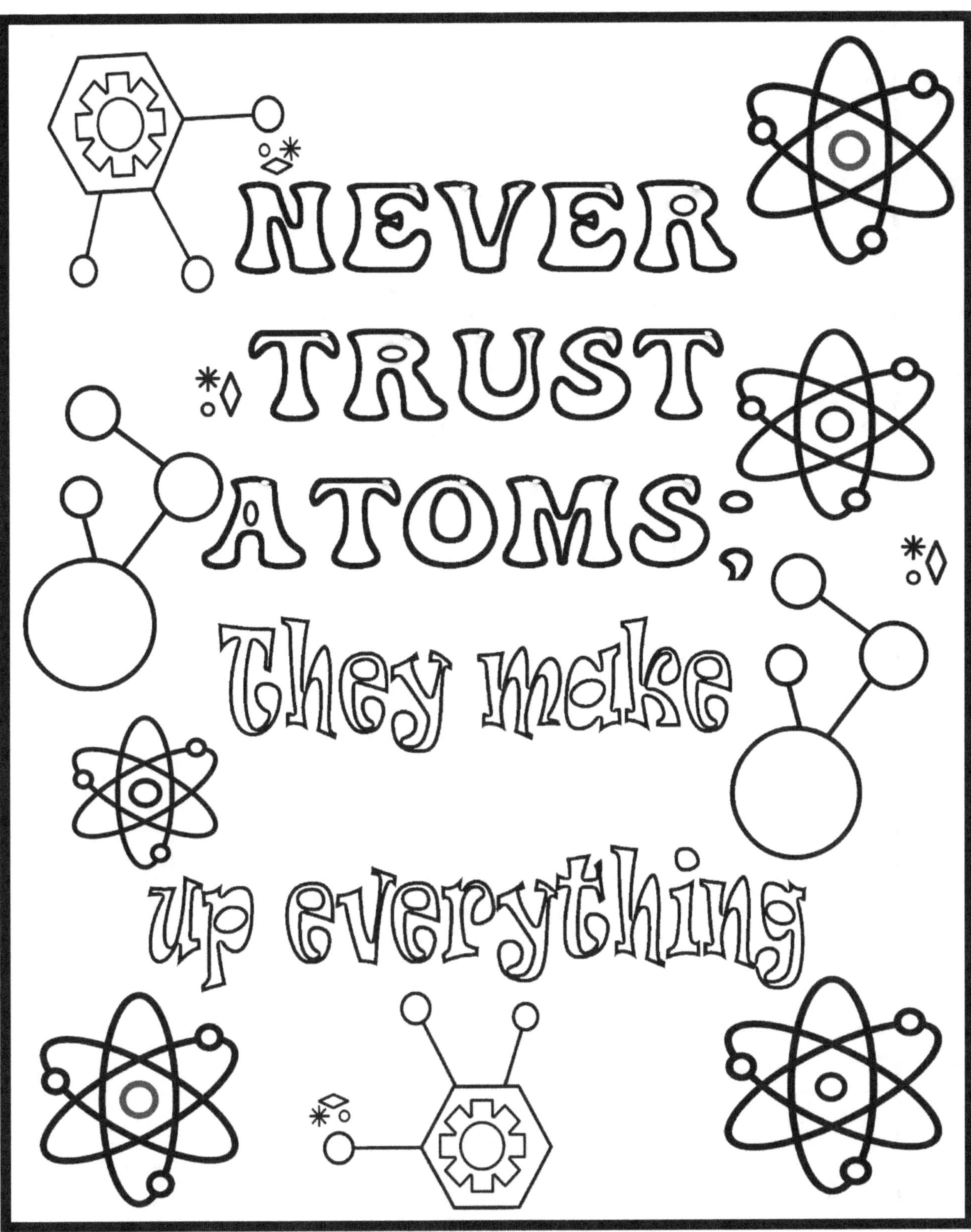

NEVER
TRUST
ATOMS,
They make
up everything

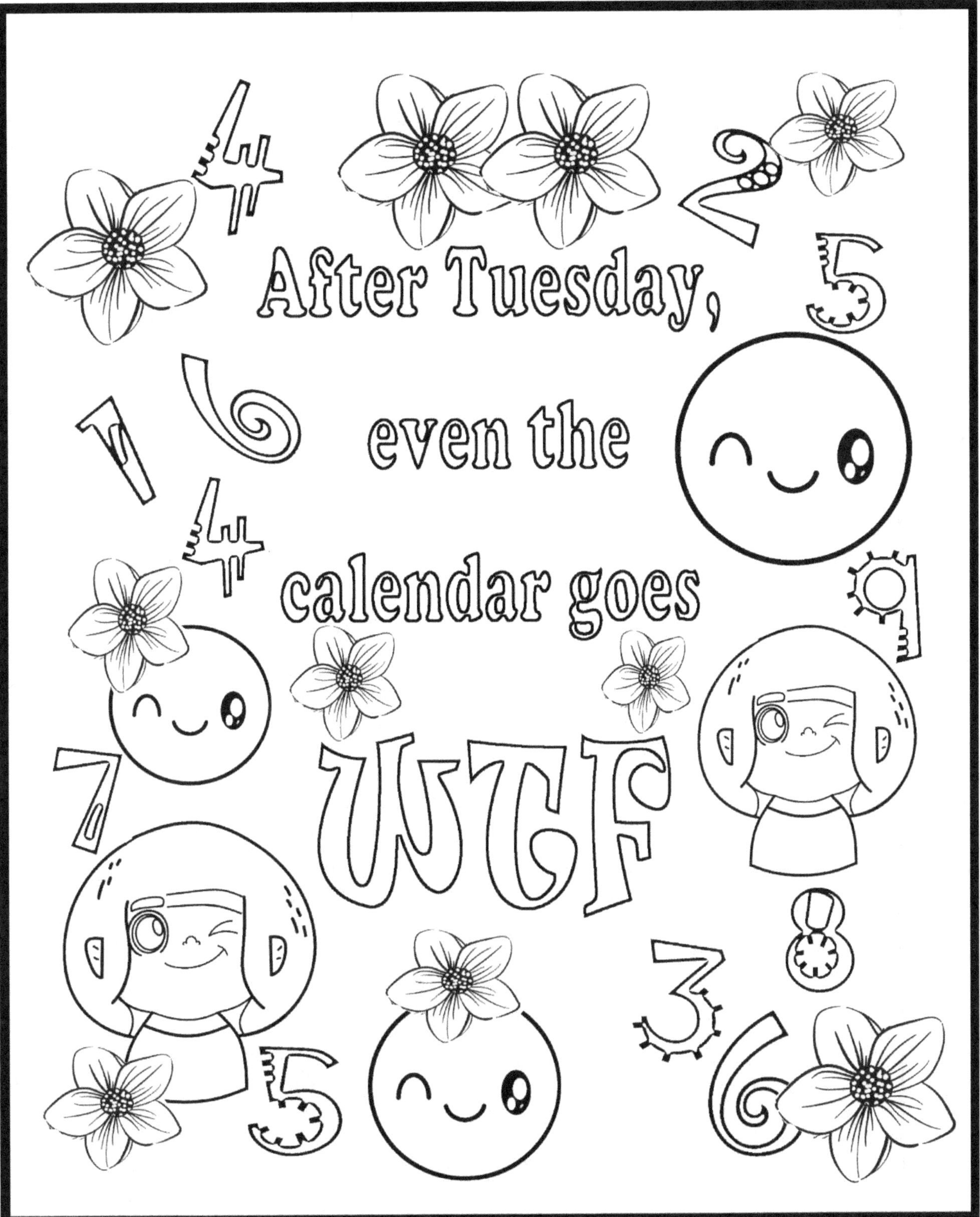
After Tuesday,
even the
calendar goes
WTF

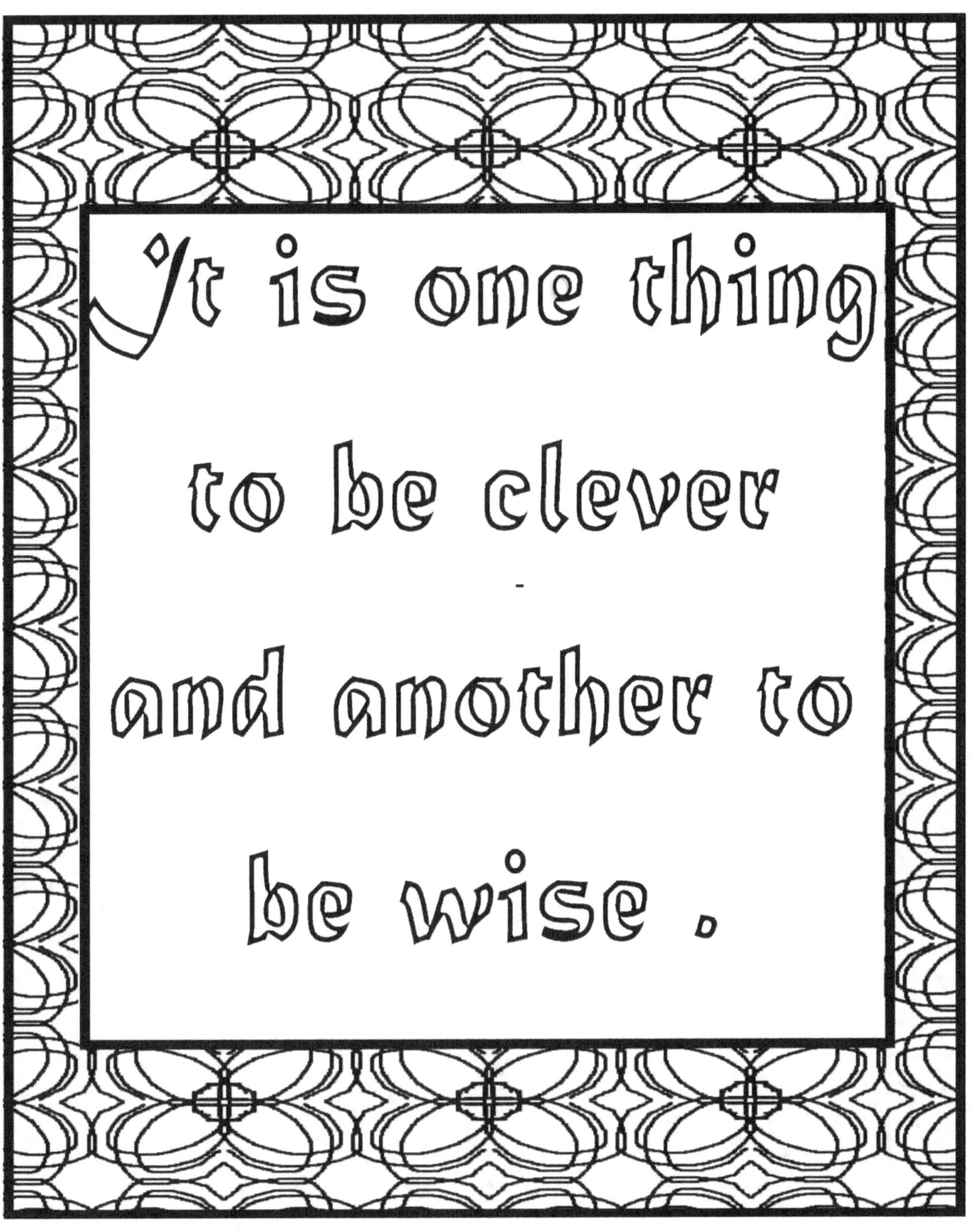
It is one thing
to be clever
and another to
be wise .

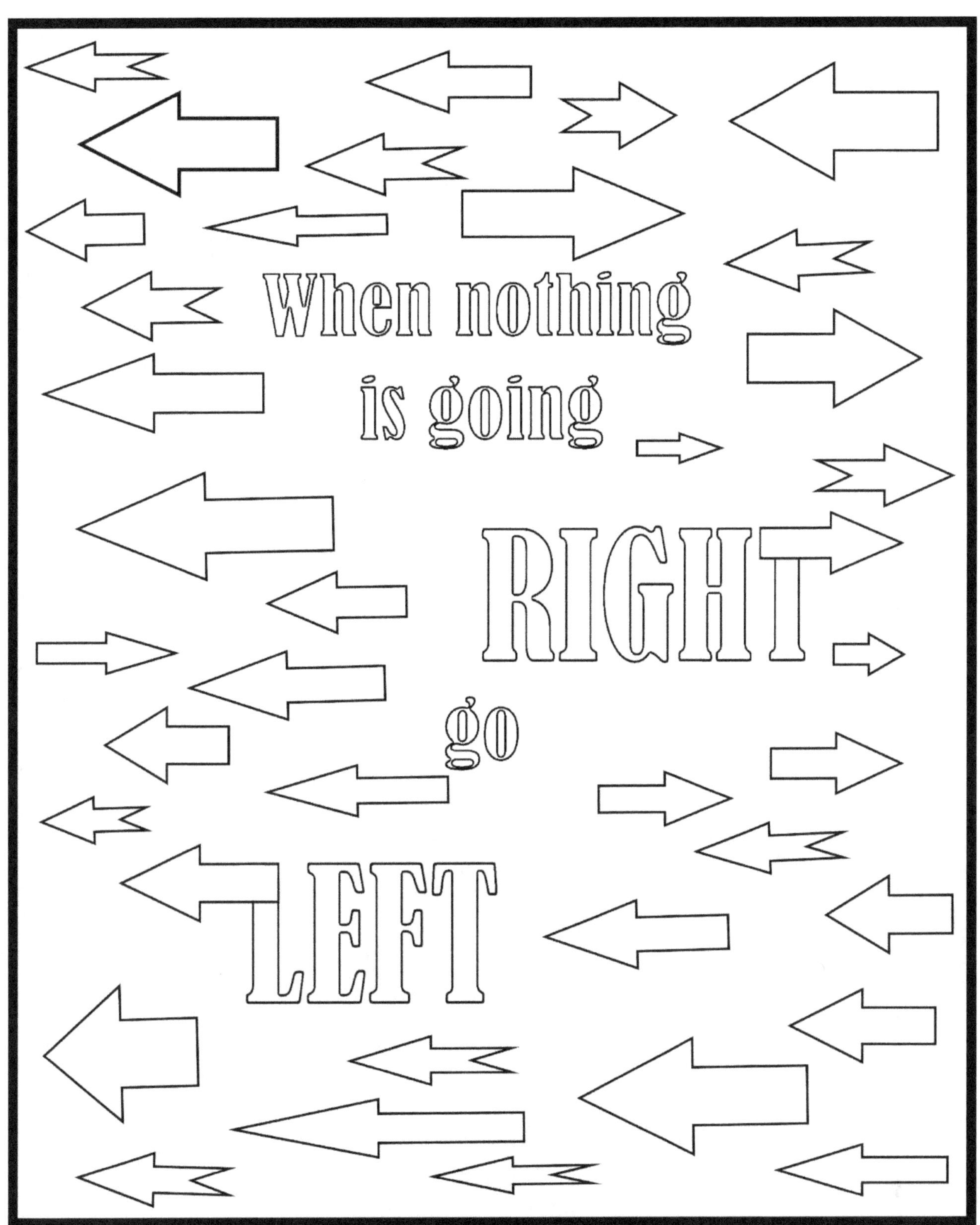

When nothing is going
RIGHT
go
LEFT

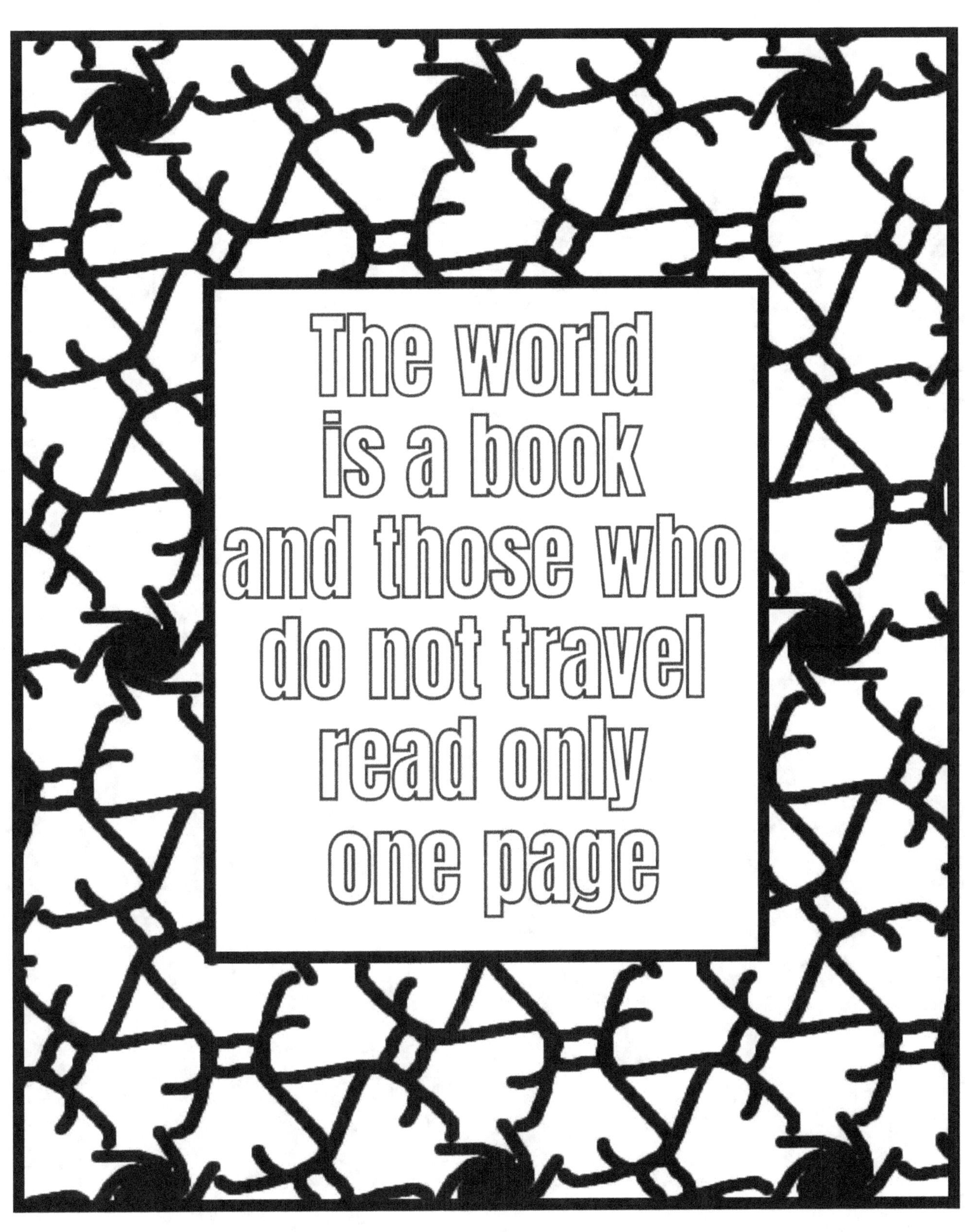
The world
is a book
and those who
do not travel
read only
one page